DEDICATION

This book is dedicated to the saga of human spirit overcoming the sufferings in life; through scientific and humanist thoughts, right attitudes and positive actions. It shares the hopes, dreams and happiness of children, youth and adults alike; to create a better and happy world.

ACKNOWLEDGEMENT

We are extremely thankful to our friends and family members, who encouraged us in bringing of this pictorial short version of our earlier book, "You must be Kidding Dr. Supratic Gupta", which covered all the topics in details. All inputs and feedbacks serve important role in strengthening the awesome rainbow of ideas, which conceived out of eventful life experiences.

We are much thankful to our family members, including our life partners, siblings, friends, Sanjoy Dasgupta, Avijit Sen and students, who helped us much in bringing out the best in us. We are also thankful to Divya Singh and Abak Saha for the designing of the book.

Authors

THE NEVER ENDING JOURNEY

The caravan of ideas on social issues rolled in slowly but firmly, rooted in Dr. Supratic Gupta's life experiences in Guwahati, Japan and Delhi. His comrade-in arms, social worker & counsellor Prakash Chandra joined him later in this mission. After four years of concerted efforts, the innovative thoughts were compiled and published in form of the book "You must be Kidding, Dr. Supratic Gupta". The intention was evidently clear, to start serious introspection on these issues, to be followed by systematic research and interventions for creating a better world. This book is designed as pictorial representation of the earlier published book. The visuals and graphics as well the out-of-box ideas are presented in a clear, concise and comprehensible way.

Indian society is undergoing a vast transformation in the social, economical and cultural values. Significant improvement has been seen in education, services, health care and other sectors. Yet, the goals of ensuring equality between rich and poor, men and women seems to be eluding. There is also a need for understanding the life and challenges of an average Indian, and take a fresh approach to the attitudes on child growth, women liberation, sports, education. research, mass entertainment and counselling.

Life passes through a series of developmental steps starting right from, birth to childhood, adolescence, schooling, college life, marriage, child birth, parenting, middle age and old age. For a balanced and happy life, there is a need to look into alternative ways of life taking reference from experiences from other countries. The book emphasises importance of pre and post birth counselling; effective child care system, swimming, flexibility exercise, music, dance, yoga and meditation. It also advocates life skill development through various counselling modules.

The journey starts from the womb; a tiny baby growing like a flower's bud. The mother needs proper training - **pre/post birth counselling**. In Japan, parents are made aware about the processes and requirements of the child growth in the womb and after birth. The **Hoikuen child care system (Japan)** is recommended so that women can carry on her job without worrying. In India the working women have to carry out double burdens - the job responsibility and the home chores. If a couple decides not to cook food at home, there is no healthy alternative food option in form of **community kitchen.**

Along with gender sensitization and unbiased environment, home management training is needed for both sex, right from very young age. **Counselling** is a type of lubricant involving guidance from a professionally trained person, which help a person pass over different stages of life, right from childhood, to adolescent, youth, adulthood, mid-age and old age. It should be compulsorily done to prepare us in each of the approaching stages of life.

This book also emphasises the importance of **mass music and dance** in life as exercise and socializing needs without bothering about individual excellence. Songs and dances are considered as types of breathing and physical exercises respectively. In addition, practicing **swimming and flexibility exercises** along with dance, music and singing from childhood would leads to proper mental and physical growth.

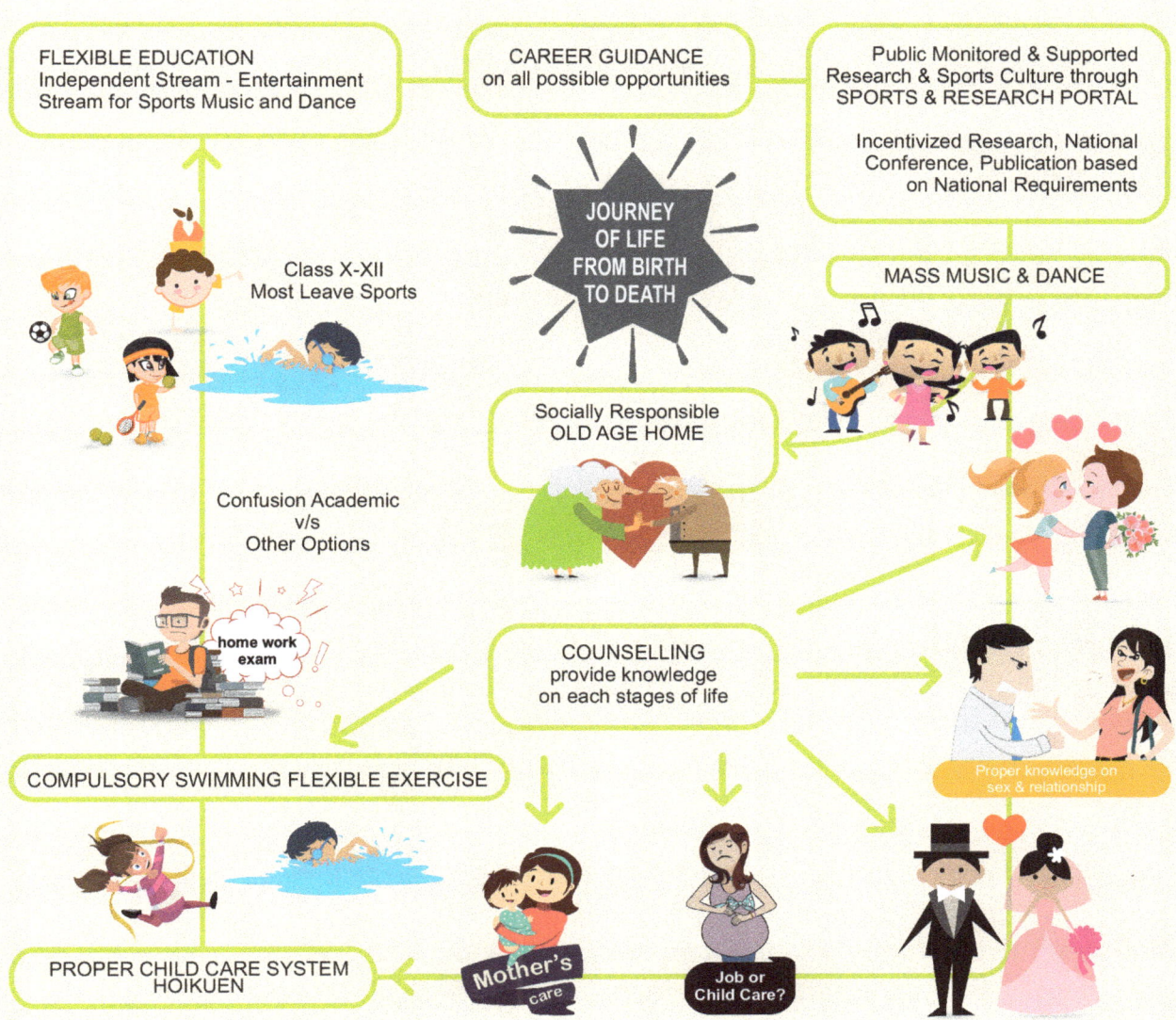

Education is another priority area for the society. The Indian government, from time to time, has taken many steps to decrease the study pressure and make it fruitful as well as enjoyable. Despite these efforts, children are still suffering under extreme study related stress. In Class IX, most children have to leave sports or physical exercise for concentrating on Board Exams. Even after completing college study, most of the students are not sure of their career goals. To address this problem, an **education portal** is proposed, where children will be made aware of all career options and job possibilities. The period for selection of specialization should be brought down to Class IX in place of class XI. An independent **entertainment stream** is also required merging the sports, music and dance.

Research culture is also important for dynamic growth of a developing country like India. The true connotation of research is introspection with systematic scientific thinking. Research applies to scientific development as well as social growth. A **research portal** with public monitoring and funding is proposed. The book also promotes **National Conference, Research Journals** as well as participation of faculties in politics.

It is proposed to carry out comparative study of the **life of women** across different regions and cultures and look at the world through their eyes. Women in cross cultural setting have different and often unique experiences regarding their growing up, sexuality, career and relationship.

LIFE IN DEVELOPING COUNTRIES

Social reformers like Swami Vivekananda have reiterated that the litmus test of society's health depends on the quality of life of women and children. The components of problems related to women and children are to be clubbed and analysed separately as well as integrally. Various attempts have been made to improve the status of children and women in different parts of the developing world. The social reforms for eradicating problems such as, child marriage, women education, dowry, inheritance for women, have largely been successful in last six decades. From very childhood, girls are brought up with lovingly by parents and often they perform much better in comparison to boys in study and activities. Now-a-days, they are participating in almost equal footings with boys, in sports and extracurricular activities. However, attaining the goals of happiness and freedom for women is still a far-fetched dream.

Modern education system and society have pushed the average age of marriage from 13-18 years to 19-30 years of age with in the last few decades. It is natural for a girl to dream of a successful career. Her biggest problem is to balance her dream with the time required for childcare, household duties and family relationships. A significant percentage of women leave jobs to take care of their children. A **strong child care system** and **community kitchen** is desirable so that women can contribute to the development of the country also.

Modern age society provides more information to the boys and girls about sex, health issues, child birth or child care in comparison to the earlier period. There is virtually an information explosion on internet and social media. But the question arises; are they getting accurate, authentic and real information relevant for the healthy development of the child?

Right from birth, the child needs to be provided right types of food with required essential nutrition. Physical exercise is also very important for proper and healthy growth. Indian parents often put over- emphasis on studies. We need to change this mind-set and provide essential trainings in swimming, flexibility exercise, song, music and dance to each and every child to create a healthy society.

Counselling is often connoted with negative sense; asking for help is still a taboo for many. We should not only promote counselling when faced with grave problems, but also utilise counselling training modules as preventive tools, so that people could anticipate the approaching problems and get equipped to face them. Most problems in life are recurring and can be learned though counselling-based modules.

Finally, as old age approaches, misery comes to many. The current old care systems are unable to address the health and other issues adequately or assure the old-aged their right to happiness. A family-based and socially responsible old age home with better facilities and health care is much needed.

COUNSELLING

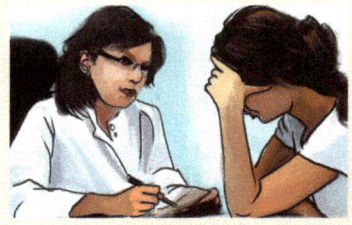
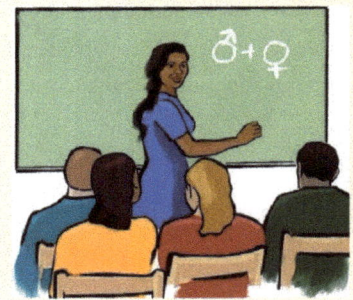
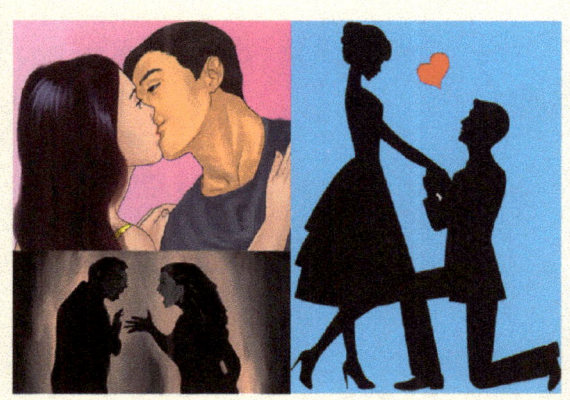
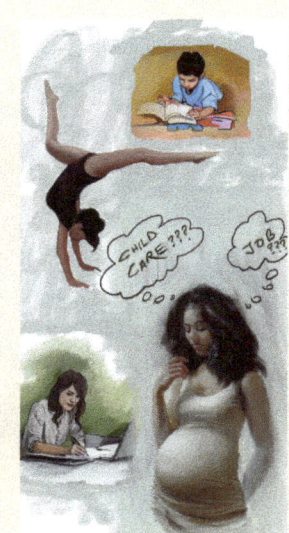

Counselling is needed in each stage of life. It is a helping tool for a person trapped in indecisive, disturbed, incongruent and stressful situations in life. Counselling can be a preventive tool too, helping people about knowing about the upcoming problems in life and learn skills to face it. It ensures guidance support and psychological help from a trained volunteer or counsellor. The importance of mental health, adjustment, coping skills, stress management and mind/anger control in Indian scenario can not be underrated.

Adolescence counselling is the need of the hour. Young boys and girls need greater gender sensitization and sexuality trainings, right from childhood to adolescence. They also needs trainings in compatibility, household chores, cooking, hygiene and physical exercises. For the marriageable youth, **Pre-Marital and Post- Marital counselling** modules have been proposed, which will make them aware about how to handle problems of maladjustment and marital discords. They have also to learn about the relationship building skills and sexual compatibility issues.

Mid life and **Old Age** are the stages of life, which requires more understanding and support. The objectives of midlife and old age counselling is to develop coping skills among the middle/old aged persons, so that they are able to face the period of psychological stress and turmoil, due to transitional special conditions. It aims to make people more aware of the concerned issues, so that they can navigate the problems in balanced and adjusting way. People have to learn to approach the void in life in better way, mentally as well as psychologically.

An **effective pre-birth** and **post- birth counselling** program is proposed, where the expectant mothers and fathers can understand the process of child development; before and after birth. It will make them equipped to handle the related challenges and problems. For children, three years of age is the most important stage of physical and mental development. The child need to develop; the immune system, the five senses, human values, healthy food habits and the interpersonal relationship.

WOMEN'S DILEMMA

National Human Resource

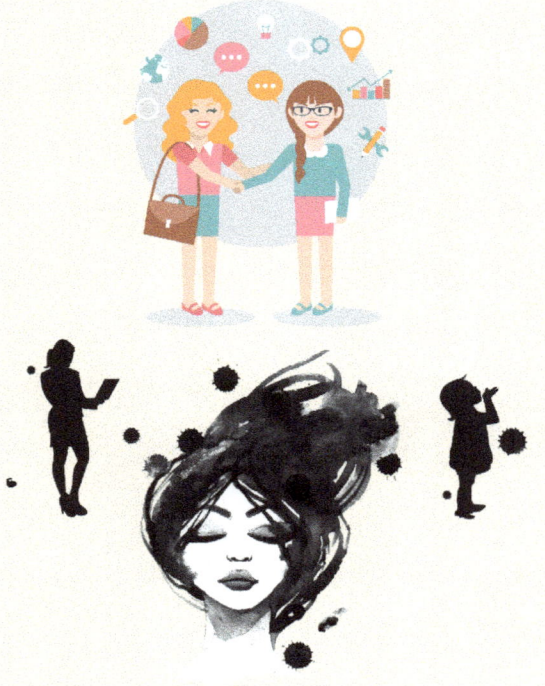

Work or Child Care

The making of career choice by girls is a difficult and complicated propositions, as they generally wish to settle down in job and marriage faster in comparison to boys. Beyonce Knowles asserts that the earning power of women is an important criterion for gender equality. But this is not an easy question, as motherhood puts them on a difficult dilemma.

Woman is always expected to be an able and efficient jugglers, carrying out the double burdens of the job responsibility as well as home chores, washing clothes and cooking food. We expect them to have ten hands of Durga and to perform like a superwoman. If a couple decides not to cook food at home, very few healthy food options are available in India. Motherhood cannot be compromised. Delayed motherhood creates more complications. It is not just the childbirth; it is the anxiety of how the child grows that keeps the women away from work place.

In the evolutionary growth of the human race, the subjugation of the women by male-dominated hierarchical society is a bitter truth. This discriminatory attitude had divided the social order, right from the earliest human civilisation. It also is linked with creating a just and happy society, where our children can grow up in a safe environment, with no sexual bias.

In the case of girls, puberty generally onsets two to three years earlier than the boys. As the girls grow faster, the inner feelings, emotions and the sexual urges often disturbs them more, mentally as well as physically. The hormonal reactions and preparation of her body for motherhood starts early. In earlier times, women married and attained motherhood in younger age. But due to significant increase in the age of marriage and job women looking for stability in careers, new problems have been created.

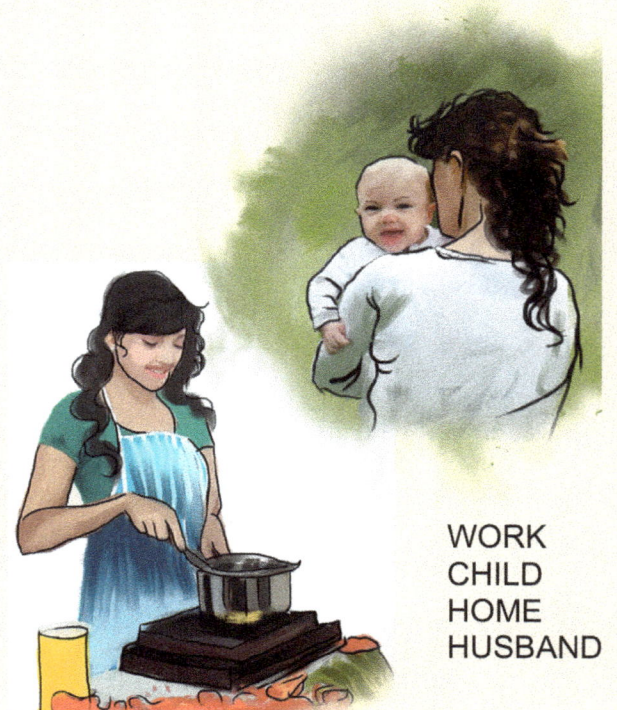

WORK
CHILD
HOME
HUSBAND

OLD AGE HOME
WITH SOCIAL RESPONSIBILITY

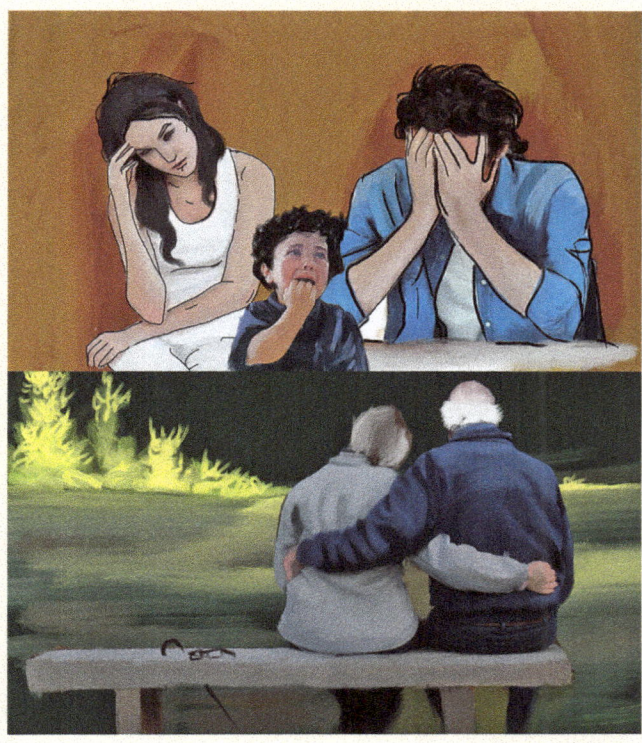

RESPONSIBLE OLD AGE
WITH SHARING OF LIFE

We tend to forget that each old person has a child struggling with in him; the child which has existed internally life long, but which has manifested fully in the old age. The child in the old person requires not only food and shelter but also needs love, care, friendship, companionship and trust. Old people like to enjoy life, laugh and sing. We need more effective alternative old age care system in India. The conditions prevailing in most of the old age homes in India are dismal. There are more than a thousand old age homes in India, including the government run centres. There is also lack of emotional and psychological support in most of the current old age homes.

A new model for a sustainable and responsible old age home is proposed and would satisfy the following:

- There are lot of nuclear families that would be benefited from nearness of the older generations as foster grand parents.
- It can also serve as an occasional childcare centre, where young parents can leave the child for quality time and mental rest.
- The people here will have lot of time. They can undertake lot of social service activities, from pre and post-birth care, counselling, etc.

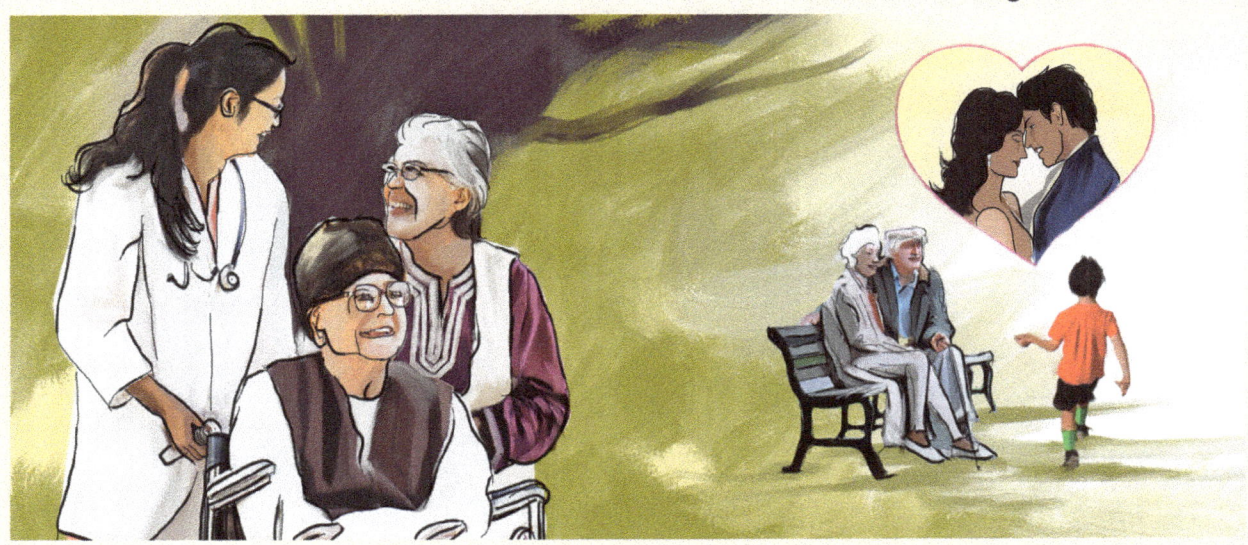

HOLISTIC CHILD CARE SYSTEM: HOIKUEN

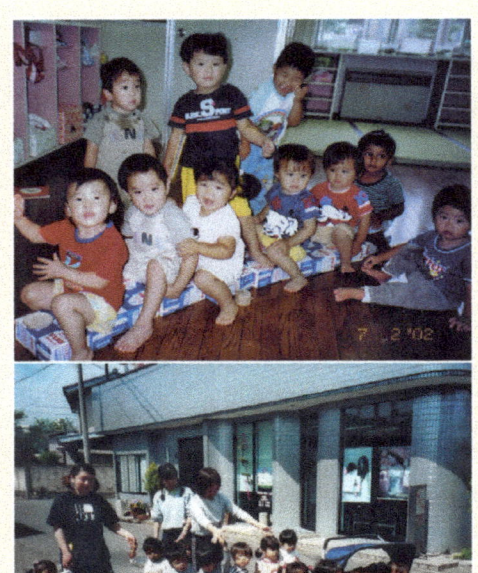

Hoikuen is the special child care system prevalent in Japan, designed to take excellent care of the children, while allowing mothers to work without worry. Unlike the traditional concept of day care, where non-trained women and domestic help take care of children; this is a complete educational system for achieving holistic development of the child. Children of working mothers can join Hoikuen even at three months of age, though usually children join it between nine and twelve months. Children continue in this system up to six years of age, after which they join regular schools.

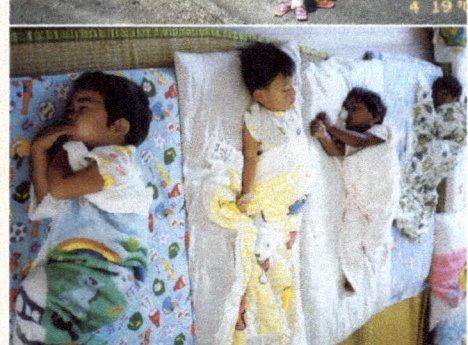

Normal Daily Life: In this system, the children arrives at very young age and learn life skills activities like; drinking, eating, sleeping, playing, interacting with each other and using toilet in a scientific way. It leads to proper and balanced personality development of the children.

Immunity: In winter and summer, children are often found playing barefoot. The children are even made to fall sick under monitored harsh conditions, so that they could develop their immune system to lead a happy and healthy adult life.

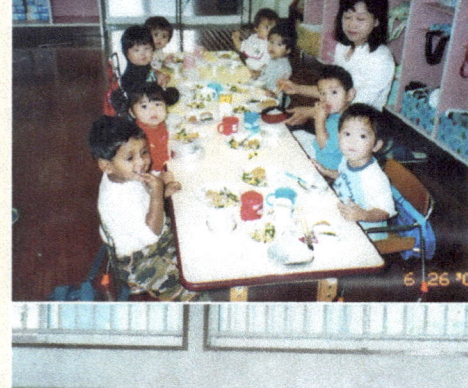

Physical and mental development: Swimming is the corner stone of physical activities in summer days. In the outdoor playground, various activities are designed in such a way that children learn balancing of the body. Music and songs also play an important role in the child development. Though formal learning through books apparently takes a backburner. Yet, by the age of six, children are well prepared to join school with much broader education. Hoikuen lays the foundation of establishing a sincere, disciplined and hardworking population that provides Japan leading edge of being a successful country.

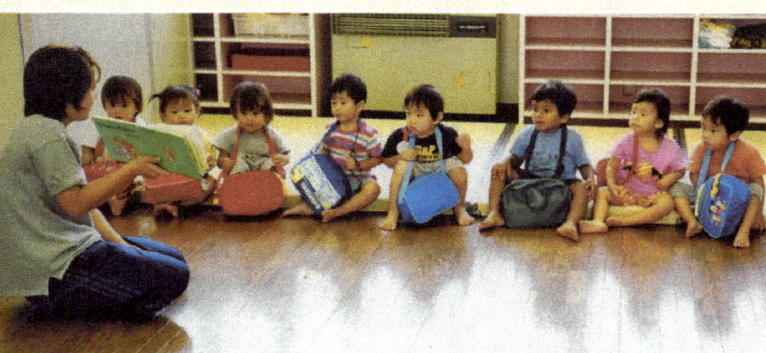

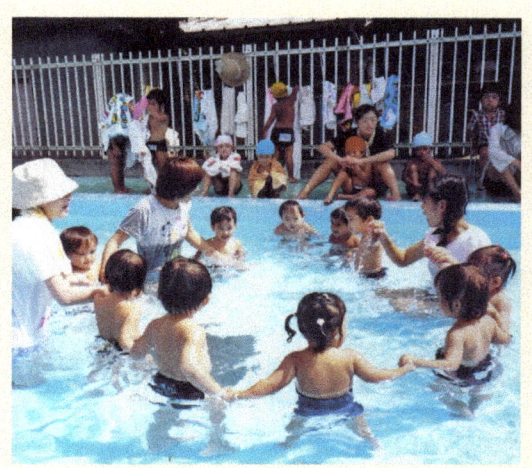

Water Activities: The physical development of children is closely linked to playing in water. We all know that the foetal baby grows in water, i.e. placenta inside the womb of the mother. Hence, babies usually love water. In Japan, children spend substantial time of the Hoikuen class in water. In home too, they are put in bathtubs along with the parents. Very small children use balloon pools, while elder children get into swimming pools. By the age of six years, most children can do synchronized swimming. They also play games of searching colour balls, shaped objects under water, which enable them to see under water.

COMMUNITY KITCHEN

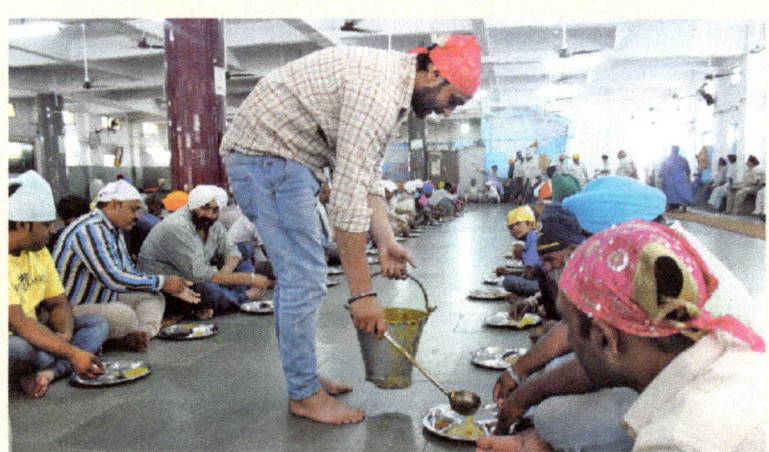

Concept of Community Kitchen : Shokudo

Cooking food is another challenge for working ladies, which makes their life hectic and tiresome. Food options available outside including restaurant and home-delivery from food chains, do not provide homely, economical and balanced food. The community kitchen is much needed to support working mothers in India. This will provide healthy choice of food in a mutually sustainable way. In India, the Langar system feeding thousands of devotees in Gurudwaras, is a type of community kitchen. IIT Madras has dismantled mess in each of the hostels and have created a combined mess providing better choice of food in a sustainable manner.

Japan has a very effective community kitchen system called Shokudo, available in most localities and residential areas. The food is cooked in various pre-fixed categories – soup, salad, main course, deserts, etc. Every day, a limited number of food options are provided and one cannot order special and separate dishes, but have to choose among the few available menu-choices. In this system, food is served quick, warm and healthy. This leads to less wastage. Countries like Germany have also adopted this system. We need to have community kitchen system available in colleges and each residential locality.

SWIMMING AND EXERCISE
IN CHILDHOOD

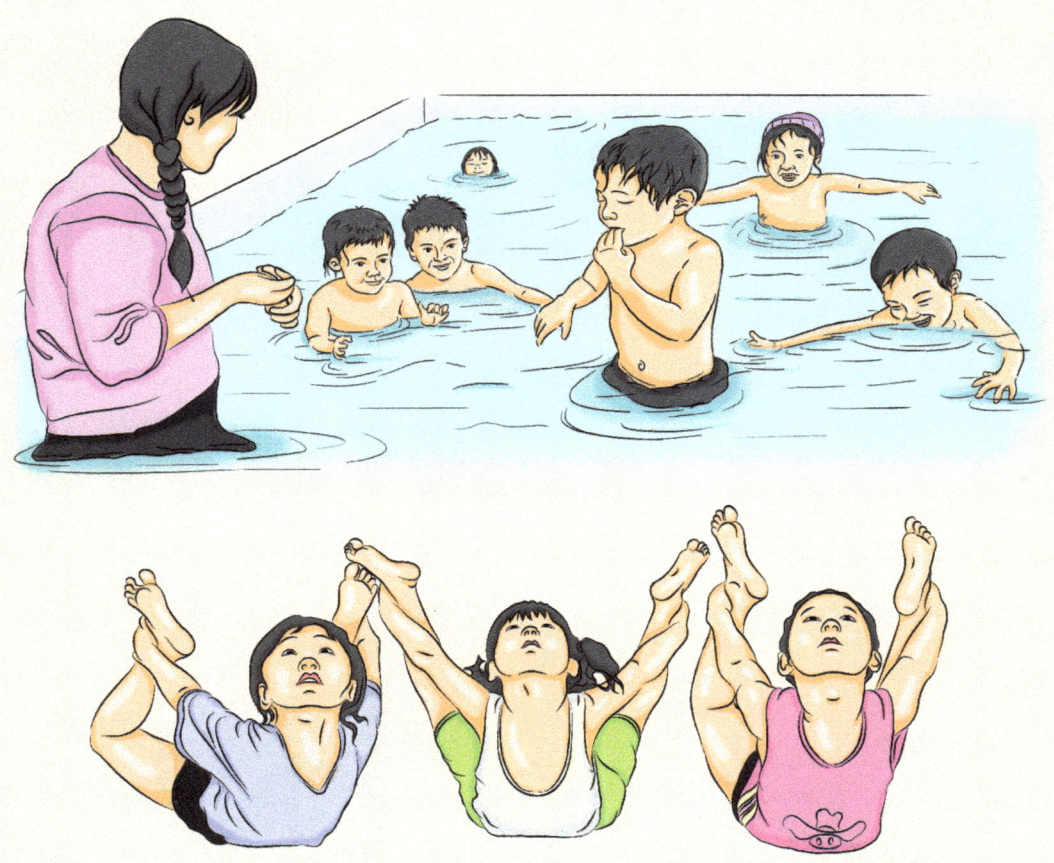

A child born today is the future asset of the country and all the energy should be dedicated to improve the health, growth and future of the child. The formative years, ranging from 0-6 years, become the foundation stone of a healthy mind in a healthy body. Flexibility exercises and water games in the formative years are very important for it.

For a baby, the movement and exercises starts at mother's womb. It approximates to swimming in the placenta fluid in the womb. In Japan, mothers make sure that the children spend substantial time of the day in water. At home, the child is put in water in bathtub along with the parents for about an hour. In Hoikuen, the children are allowed water games. Activities are designed to build up the flexibility, stamina, strength and balance, for mental and physical growth among children, such that sensory perception, motor skills, social relationship skills are developed.

Countries like Japan gives high priority to flexibility and floor exercises for the small children. Importance is being given to gymnastics, which is considered as the foundation and mother of all other sports. It develops a healthy and flexible body. South American countries lay special emphasis of dance in their life, which makes their body extremely healthy and flexible. China and Japan have taken the path of martial arts. The possibility of implementing flexibility exercise from childhood along with yoga, pranayama, floor exercise, martial arts, etc. need to be explored. Collaborations with these countries is required in future.

MASS MUSIC AND DANCE

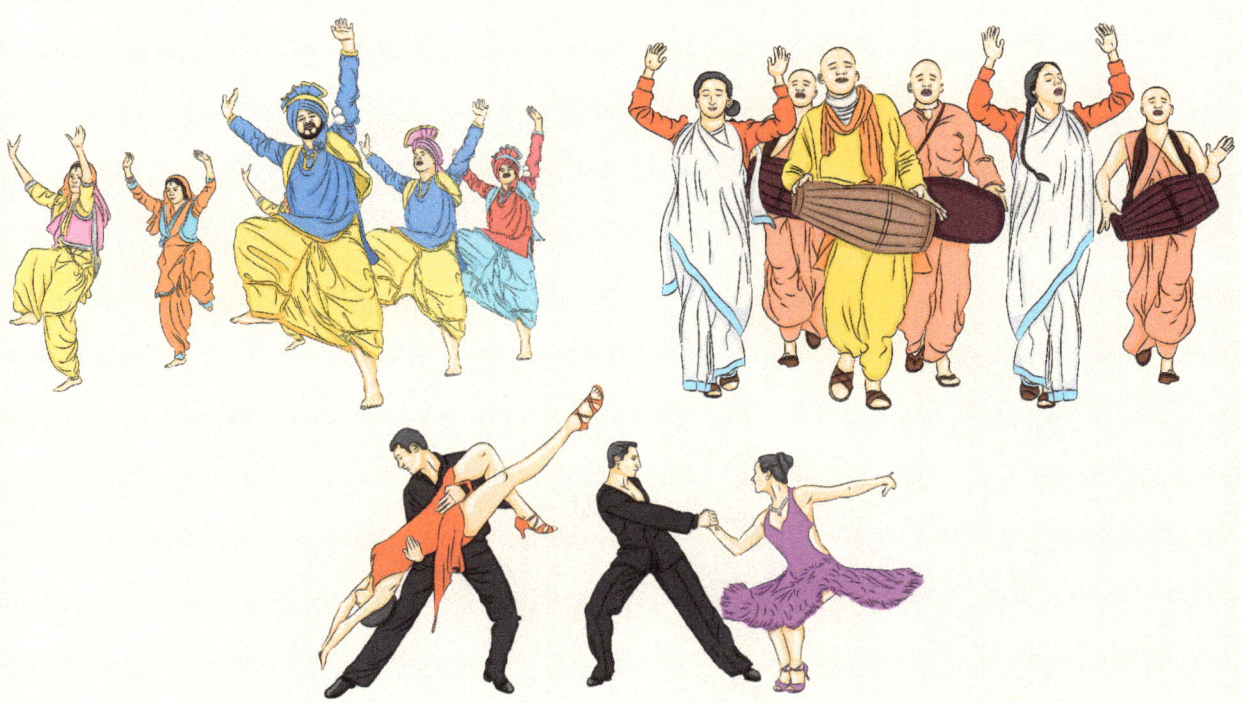

Singing, music and dance are corner stones of happiness in any society. It is a strong medium of communication. Practice of singing provides better breathing practice, while music provides us a sense of rhythm and dance provides us a flexible and healthy body. Different religions and cultures of the world have attempted to utilise dance and music to provide a good foundation for happy society. It can be seen that all these activities are carried out in a mass participatory mode. Tribal group dances, Punjabi Bhangra dance, ISKON's Samkirtana, Art of Living's sessions, Choirs of Church and Kirtans in temples are some examples of the effective implementation of mass music and dance.

In India, usually the children are allowed to learn singing, music and dance on individual basis. Singing, music and dance are seen as artistic and extracurricular activities, practised only by talented children. Most children find it difficult to sustain the practice in long terms and the dropout rate is high. Most of people enjoy hearing song, but only few venture to perform it in public audience, due to being shy and hesitant. We propose to strengthen this culture of participative mass music and dance, so that they can become an integrated part and parcel of our society. Japanese Karaoke system is a great system, which when played in a closed enclosure provides us great opportunity to sing loudly. Aerobics, Jumba, Salsha are great forms of dance worth learning. We need to realize that people should participate in singing, music and dance, without any inhibitions and hesitation. It creates a happy and vibrant socialization and mass relaxation.

An experiment was conducted at IIT Delhi, where about 150 students danced Jumba under the able guidance of trained instructors from Delhi Dance Academy. It was called "Dancercise"– a term coined by Madhuri Dixit, meaning Dance as Exercise. This experiment was a great success.

EDUCATION SYSTEM IN INDIA

In comparison to other countries, Indian education system is putting undue emphasis on formal education. It appears that we are still carrying the outdated legacy of Lord Macualay's education system of 19th century. This disturbs development of skills in other fields of business, music, dance, sports, etc., which has much larger social need. The existing system is creating great stress on the young students:

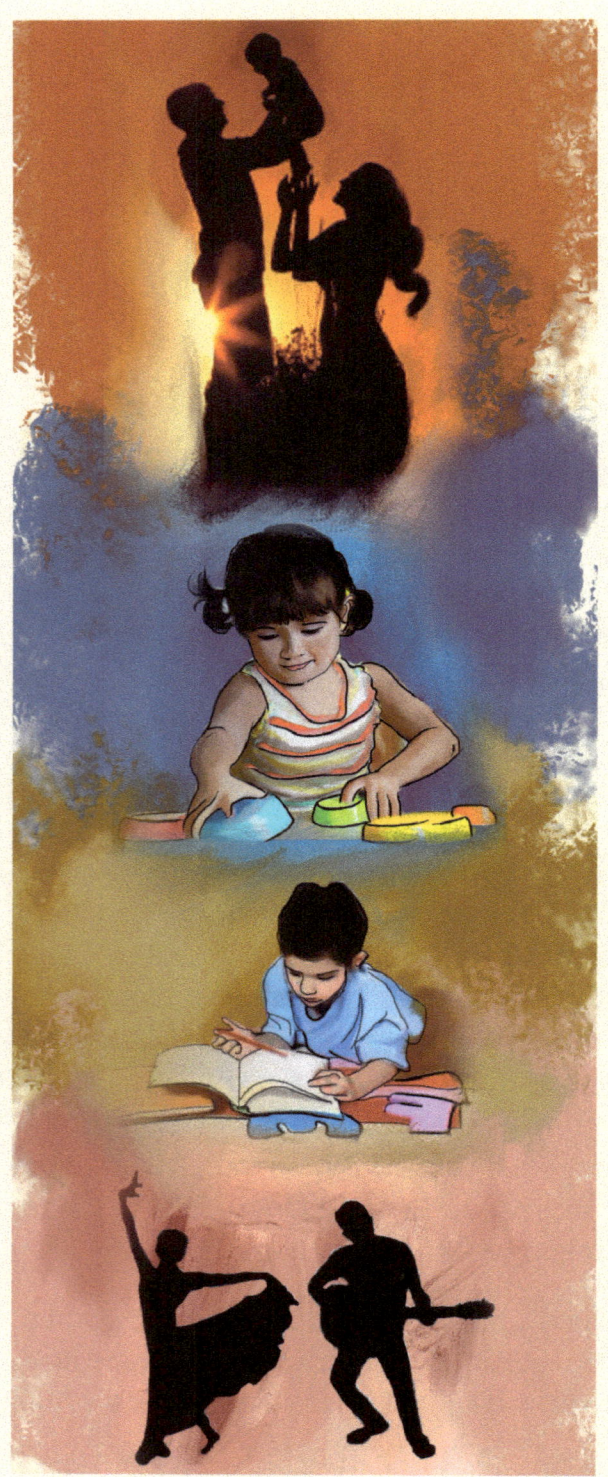

Pre-School Child Care System (0 – 3 years): The initial years of child care are mostly in the hand of mothers. It is assumed generally that a mother's instinct knows best, how to take care of the child. In case of working mothers, the children are either taken care by grandparents, nanny (often untrained) or in a child care home or crèche. Unfortunately, in India, this is one of the most neglected sectors, with shabby places, untrained & underpaid caretakers and lack of childcare experts.

Pre-primary system (3-6 years): The present Indian education system starts at age the age of 3-4 years, with pre-primary system. Most of the times, these schools are built in cramped buildings, claiming to follow Montessori or other modern teaching methodologies. But the fact is that, majority of them lack good quality and trained primary teachers. There is often no space for playground or scope of flexibility exercises. Learning the alphabets, rhymes, drawing and singing becomes the primary goal.

Primary and Middle School System (Class 1 to VIII): This is supposed to be the most enjoyable part of the life. Parents want their children to perform well in studies as well as indulge in some extra-curricular activities like music, dance, art, games, etc. As the child grows, there is extreme pressure due to study and interests/hobby. The children having special background, e.g. from business back ground or with parents from sports, dance and music back ground are luckier to get appropriate training necessary to be successful in such trade of life.

Secondary School (Class IX and X): This is the most critical pubertal stage of life for physical growth of the boys and girls. An excellent atmosphere for sports would have created a strong body, great endurance and stamina. But unfortunately, at this stage, our education system emphasises on the academic performance. The latent energy of the children in sports, music and dance are suppressed as they are forced to concentrate on their study.

Higher Secondary School (Class XI and XII): In our current educational system, the child has to take one of the most important decisions of the life – selection between science, arts and commerce stream. Once the decision is taken, there is no much chance of changing stream afterwards, even when the children performance is poor in the selected stream. Many children drop out and join vocational diploma courses. Students who joined science, then face the next race of life: medical, engineering, or normal graduation courses.

College and Higher Education: Parents have infinite expectations with their children in performing well in the studies without bothering about the interest and aptitude of the student or about the earning capability of those streams. In fact, most of the children have no idea about the different type of jobs possible as career choices. It is at later stage that they realize that they are in a job that they do not enjoy. A typical case of Civil Engineering Department at one of the IITs says that in 2015-16, there was 80% students received job through campus placement. The rest possibly did not opt for placement through the institute for different reasons like joining services like IAS, IES or for doing MBA. Among those placed, only one was placed in core sector. To this is really sad and is possibly created due to the basic incompatibility of knowledge and expectation between the students and companies.

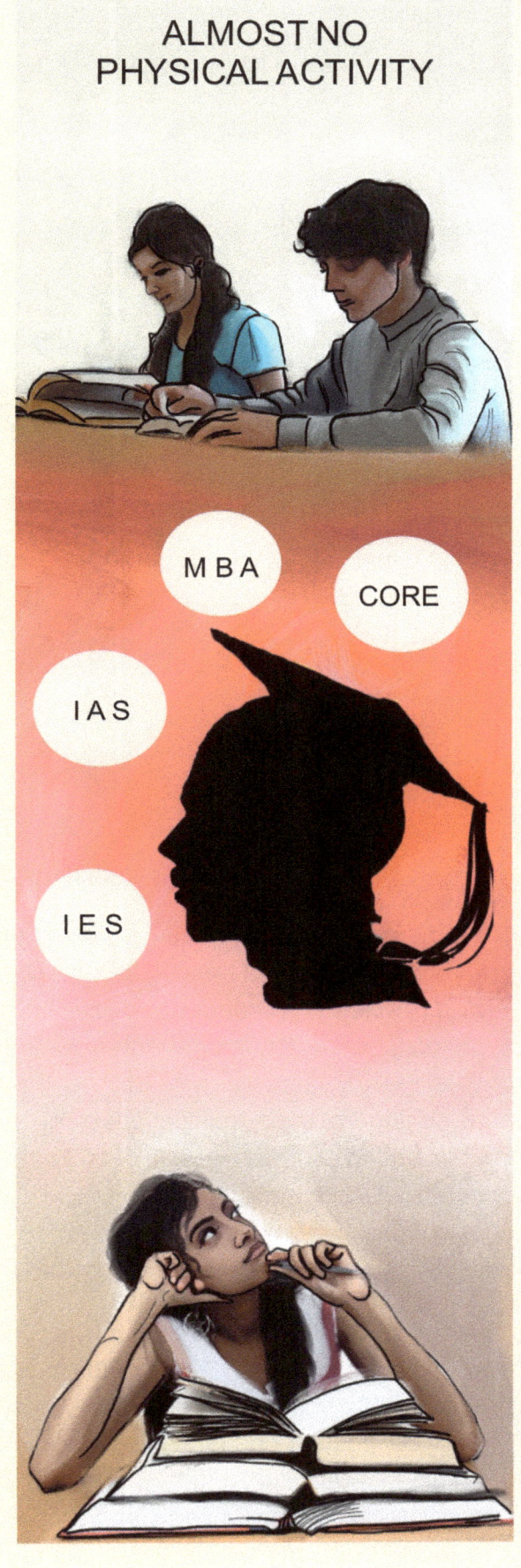

ALMOST NO PHYSICAL ACTIVITY

MBA CORE IAS IES

MODIFICATIONS NECESSARY FOR
EDUCATION SYSTEM

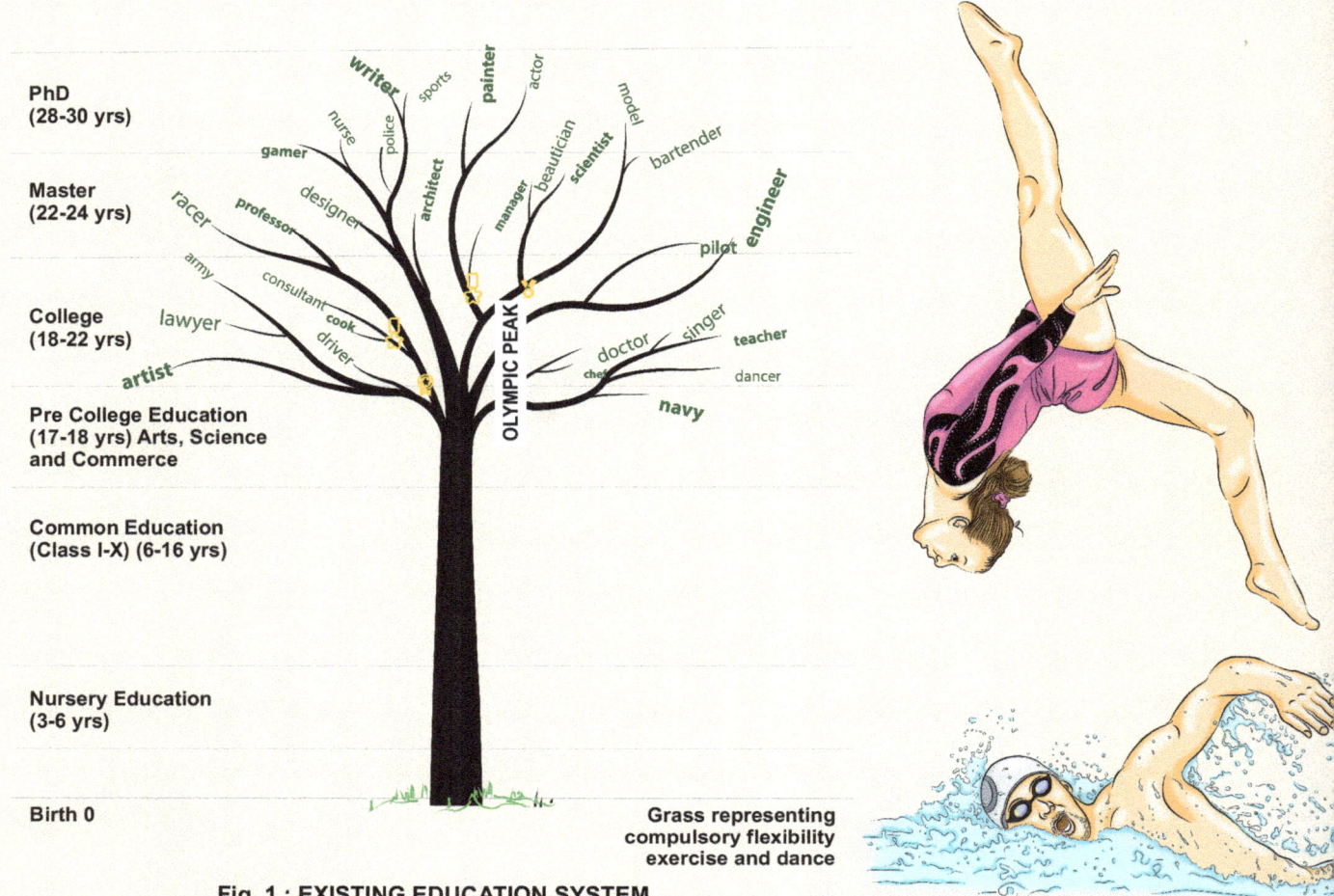

PhD
(28-30 yrs)

Master
(22-24 yrs)

College
(18-22 yrs)

Pre College Education
(17-18 yrs) Arts, Science
and Commerce

Common Education
(Class I-X) (6-16 yrs)

Nursery Education
(3-6 yrs)

Birth 0

Grass representing
compulsory flexibility
exercise and dance

Fig. 1 : EXISTING EDUCATION SYSTEM

Swimming, flexibility exercise, yoga, singing, and dance are very important for the mental and physical growth of the children, as represented by the grass in the bottom in the figure. We need scientific guidance to be provided compulsorily to all children. Hoikuen Child care system needs to be implemented so that women have the liberty to join their job. The children will be benefited as they will be brought up in the hands of trained mothers, contributing to their holistic development of mind and body. Children select line of specialization of stream at age of 16 years, which has to be lowered to age of 14 years. The children will get more time to pursue their specialization subjects, and they can even change stream. The pubertal age energy of the boys will be utilized, as the relaxed four years of course would allow them to lead a balanced life in studies, sports and exercise.

India has potential to become a sports power house. Children can choose the line of sports from early age. Sports, Music and dance requires long hours of training and dedicated practice from childhood. This often conflicts with the studies and the children suffer. Moreover, life in sports is expensive, as nutrition requirement and other equipment costs are high. In most cities and towns, large number of children are already practicing sports. It is important to do something and create an independent, self-sustained education system so that children can join this stream without inhibition.

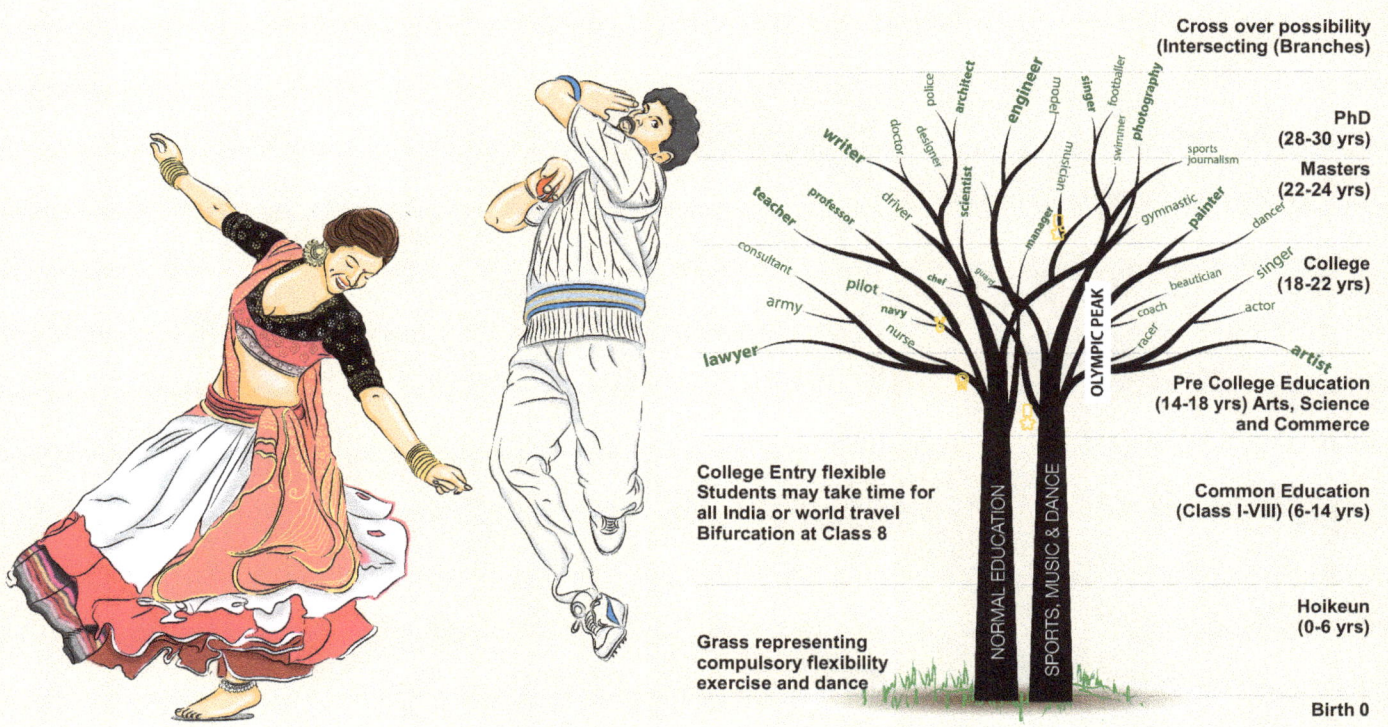

Fig. 2 - PROPOSED EDUCATION SYSTEM

Labels within figure:

Cross over possibility (Intersecting (Branches)

PhD (28-30 yrs)

Masters (22-24 yrs)

College (18-22 yrs)

Pre College Education (14-18 yrs) Arts, Science and Commerce

Common Education (Class I-VIII) (6-14 yrs)

Hoikeun (0-6 yrs)

Birth 0

College Entry flexible Students may take time for all India or world travel Bifurcation at Class 8

Grass representing compulsory flexibility exercise and dance

NORMAL EDUCATION

SPORTS, MUSIC & DANCE

OLYMPIC PEAK

writer, teacher, consultant, army, pilot, navy, nurse, lawyer, professor, driver, chef, doctor, designer, police, scientist, architect, engineer, musician, manager, singer, model, japou, swimmer, footballer, photography, sports journalism, gymnastic, painter, dancer, beautician, singer, coach, actor, racer, artist

Many of these children had to sacrifice their childhood for long practice. The star gymnast, Nadia Comaneci of Romania, Criketer Kapil Dev, Olympic Gold medallists Michel Phelps and most sports person have started their sports life early. Michel Phelps used to consume food loaded with 18000 calories per day, almost 8 times of an average person consumption. Deepika Padukone, famous Indian actress, had a hectic early morning badminton practice, tiring day school and a rigorous evening practice of Bharat Natyam dance.

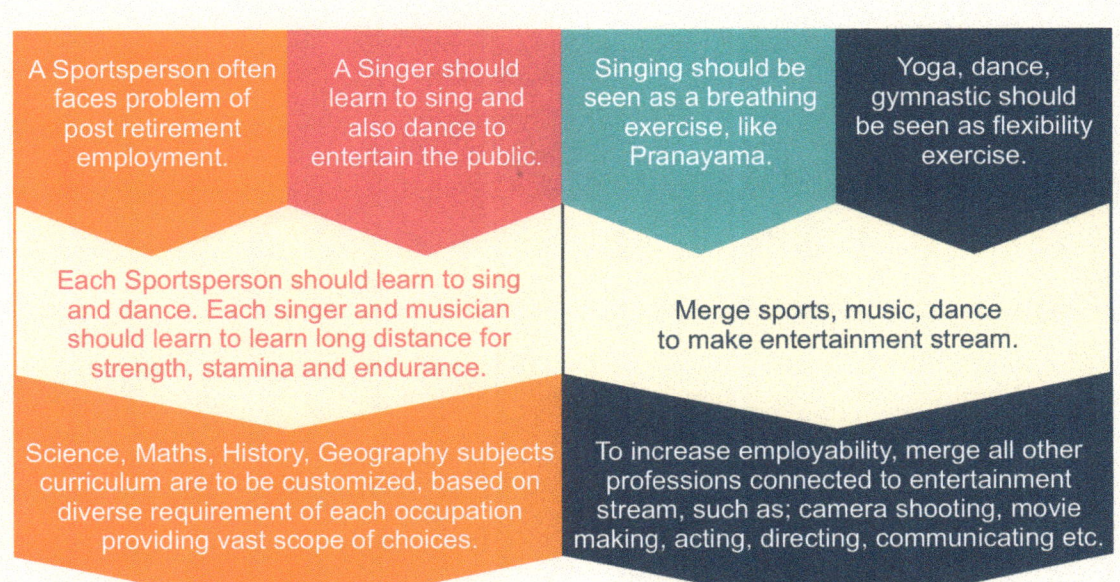

A Sportsperson often faces problem of post retirement employment.

A Singer should learn to sing and also dance to entertain the public.

Singing should be seen as a breathing exercise, like Pranayama.

Yoga, dance, gymnastic should be seen as flexibility exercise.

Each Sportsperson should learn to sing and dance. Each singer and musician should learn to learn long distance for strength, stamina and endurance.

Merge sports, music, dance to make entertainment stream.

Science, Maths, History, Geography subjects curriculum are to be customized, based on diverse requirement of each occupation providing vast scope of choices.

To increase employability, merge all other professions connected to entertainment stream, such as; camera shooting, movie making, acting, directing, communicating etc.

EDUCATION PORTAL

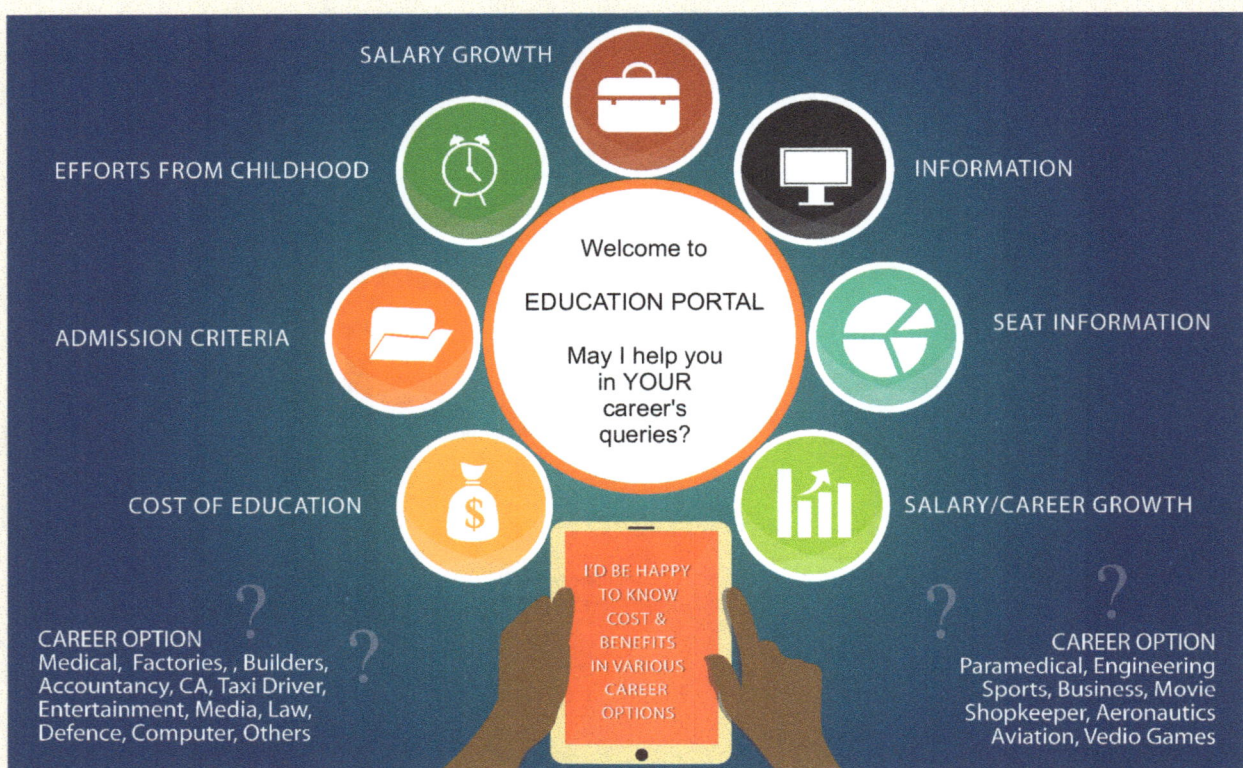

The middle class forms a substantial chunk of population in our country, which is primarily consisting of the formal job sectors and professional classes. The primary aim of middle class is to first get education and then get a job. The journey of a middle class Indian from childhood to adulthood is a pathetic story of constant race for achievement. From the very childhood, a typical child faces the competition of learning alphabets, memorizing points, learning dozens of subjects and mugging up for exams. After education, he is immediately forced to take up jobs, marriage, have children and then again work for education and career of the children.

Even in this age of internet and information explosion on career choices, youth get confused about how to select a course. So there is a need of providing web-based portal or platform, which provides qualitative information about traditional and non-traditional jobs, vocations and careers.

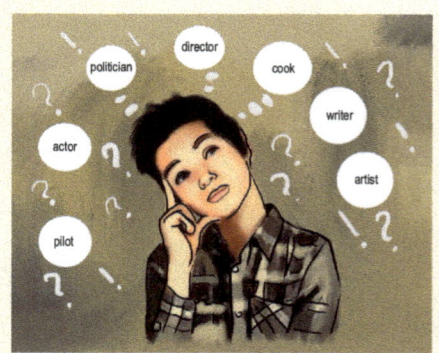

• General public and students will get access to various options relating to education and career matters on a wide platform.

• Active Participation in the portal will create more awareness among the public to take informed decisions on careers.

• The interactive portal will also satisfy the queries of the students from the experts.

• The portal will be based on a sustainable fees and subscription based model, where revenues will also be generated, from both users and advertisers.

Do I have right to choose profession of my choice?

How much will I earn?

Why do people not give equal respect to all jobs?

SELF-SUSTAINED SPORTS PORTAL

PUBLIC MONITORED SPORTS CULTURE

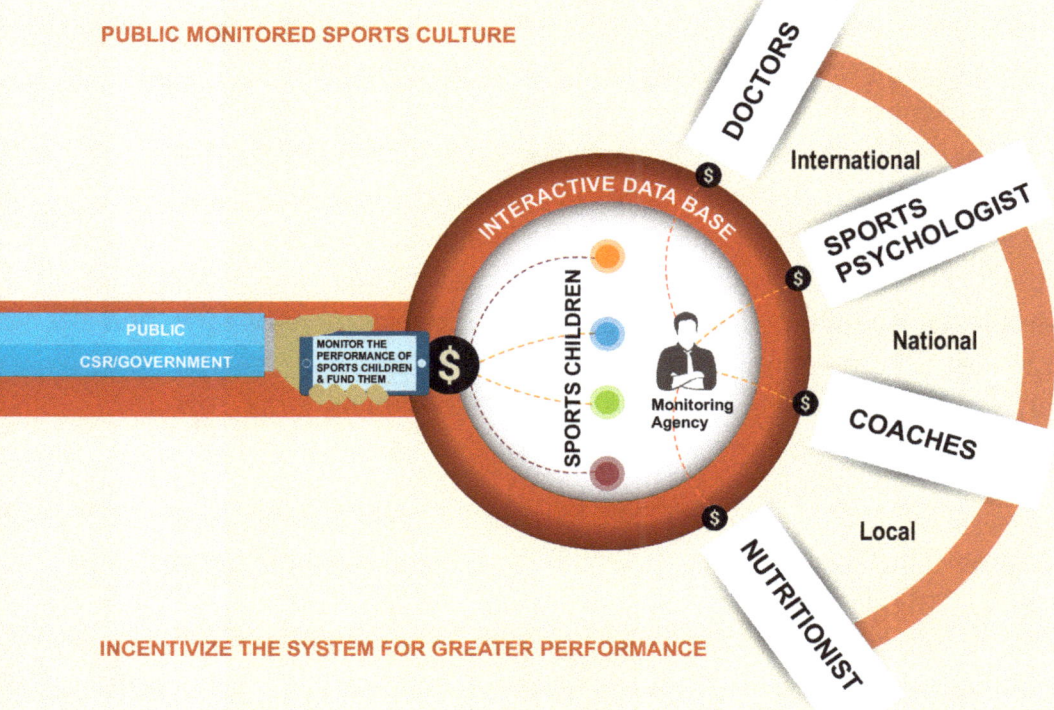

INCENTIVIZE THE SYSTEM FOR GREATER PERFORMANCE

- Continuous monitoring of activities of sports participants and creating accountability.
- Self-review of body movements, realization of training errors and comparison with other professionals.
- Evaluation by national and international experts to form the distance guidance system.
- Source of entertainment for paid readers and a source of information for new sports person.
- This will serve as a platform, where sports persons will be getting proper evaluation and individuals, companies and government can decide to sponsor them.
- Beneficiary to pay either by themselves or by sponsorship.
- Sponsors can evaluate whom they are sponsoring and evaluate their performance.
- Information related to physical development with age, correct food habits, exercise etc.

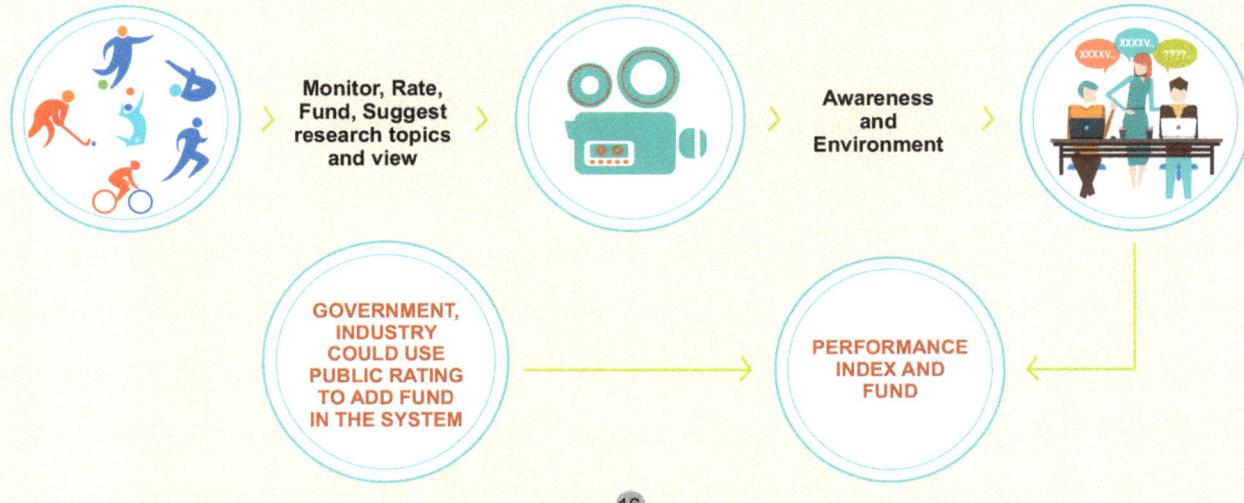

RESEARCH ENVIRONMENT IN INDIA

Any modern society would require sincere research, analysis and introspection in all human and scientific fields to grow and excel. A typical researcher identifies the problems, its objectives and tries to analyse and address the problem from a newer perspective, with an aim of creating a better world. Most of the researches are done in universities and colleges. Students undertakes research mostly to earn degree and the faculty guides the students formally. The research and education is highly subsidized by the government funds. It is expected that this research held would benefit the country and the world for the betterment of the environment, society, economy and scientific developments. Japan and USA have paid bright students from their country and world wide to come to their country and carry out research and have reaped rich dividends by implementing fertile research environment. India needs to understand these basics to be able to improve.

In India, research is being carried out in all universities to award degree of undergraduate, master and doctoral degree. Thesis work exists in each on the degrees. As per University grant Commission report 2013-14, there were 20 universities and 500 colleges with 2.1 lakhs student during independence. The number has gone up from to 666 universities, 39671 colleges and 237.65 lakhs of which 44% were women. Of these 85.12% students were undergraduate, 12.35% were post graduate and 1.68% were diploma or certificate courses and 0.85% were doing research possibly indicating doctoral studies. The number of PhD awarded were only 20275 in the year 2012-13. If one look at the situation in IIT Delhi, as per Times of India report, 1880 students graduated of which 770 were undergraduate student, 889 in post graduate level and 221 Phd students in the year 2015 [2]. The national average stands at 0.085% in comparison to 11.7% of IIT Delhi needs to be improved for the progress of the country.

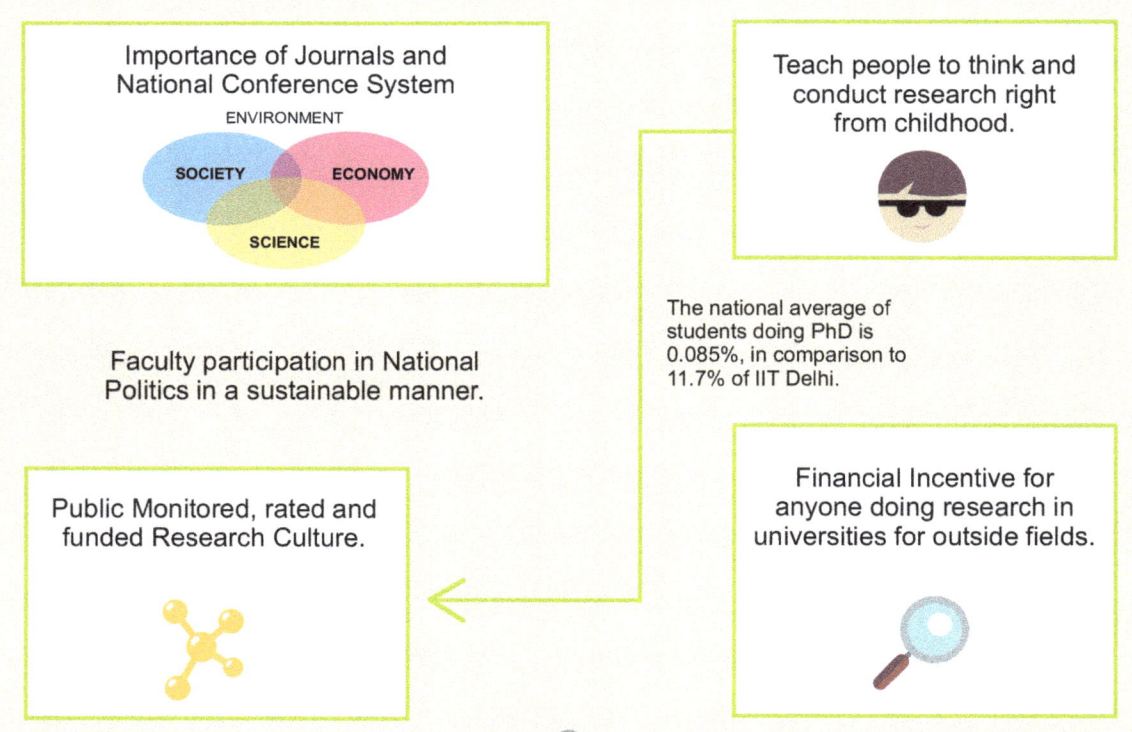

Importance of Journals and National Conference System

ENVIRONMENT

SOCIETY ECONOMY

SCIENCE

Teach people to think and conduct research right from childhood.

Faculty participation in National Politics in a sustainable manner.

The national average of students doing PhD is 0.085%, in comparison to 11.7% of IIT Delhi.

Public Monitored, rated and funded Research Culture.

Financial Incentive for anyone doing research in universities for outside fields.

Journals

Developed countries have their own well established systems of reputed journals, being published in all subjects, fields and professional areas. But in India, there is dearth of good quality and internationally accepted journals. Researchers prefer to publish their research work in international journals located in developed countries. These publications are mostly for evaluation of the researchers for their promotion purpose, rather than for the betterment of society that provides financial grants to support the research. If one looks from a different perspective, this research is mostly funded by public money. Most of these research journals are expensive and are out of bound on normal public. It is very important that the results of research carried out in India should be made accessible by the government to the public and the local industry with reasonable cost. Wherever possible, we should implement our national journals.

National Conferences

Conferences are specialized meetings where researchers are expected to publish their work and interact with each other. It is an event, where industry and interested people would be able to access the research results easier and share their experiences which will broaden their thinking-zone.

In India, most conferences are not national in character. Most of the time, research groups and institutions organize conference for their publicity and promotions. The participation are restricted and not representative of their sector's national presence. This is true for most cases, except in few sectors, where genuine National Conferences are held with wide participation. Author strongly proposes establishment of a national Conference system in which all research of particular field meet once a year. This conference should be rotated through out the country. Industry and academia interaction should increase.

Case Study - Japan

Let us take the case of societies in Civil Engineering Department in Japan. Japanese Society of Civil Engineers (JSCE) and Japan Concrete Institute (JCI) are well established and self-ustained. These organizations also get government grants, but mostly sustain themselves by the earning from membership fees and selling the journals. These organizations have their own journals and hold periodic national and international conferences. The faculty, students and professionals working in private companies are members to these organizations, making these societies financially self-sustained.

The annual conferences are attended by all students and faculty of the country in the specialization and most concerned companies also put demonstration booths to sponsor these conferences. The industry can also select bright students for employment from these conferences. These conferences are rotated through out the country. These conferences become big economic event for the city and also serves the purpose of national integration. The conference dates are such selected that master and undergraduate students doing research can each year submit their research findings here.

HOW TO THINK, WRITE DOCUMENTS AND MAKE PRESENTATION

Author has presented a new process of thinking and called it Scientific thinking to help us approach life in a organized way. This is based of approach usually adopted on research activities. Any issue or problem or phenomenon has to be approached with a structured thinking consisting of four steps - Objective, Literature Review, Content and Conclusion. In research, students are taught to write thesis in a structured manner. This is presented here and can also be followed to write any document. The thesis starts with an Introduction which explains the background of the problem, the issues, objectives and limitations. This is followed by chapters for Literature review, Theory and Experimental setup. This is followed by Content chapters representing the work done and finally the Conclusion. It is emphasised that graphical or pictorial representation to be of great importance. We also need to learn to make slides. We need to practice and learn how to present our work in short, within provided time limit. It is important to understand the knowledge level, expectations and mental status of the listener before making the presentation. While answering question and answer, we need to realized that it is not necessary to be able to answer all question.

It is important to introduce research in the lives of common people.

Common people must be trained for scientific thinking.

After this, people must be encouraged to think critically on a variety of topics.

OBJECTIVE OF THE WORK

v

LITERATURE/LIFE/FIELD REVIEW

v

ACTUAL BODY OF WORK

v

CONCLUSION

Honorarium to Faculty in Projects

In India, research is mostly sponsored by the Government. It may be an exaggeration, but researchers conduct research mostly to satisfy their academic promotion requirements. Hence, most of the time it is witnessed that, it is only the young researchers that apply for the research grant. This is mainly because Indian Government does not give honorarium for research work. Without incentive, the system does not work. Non-provision of honorarium also encourages the possibility of false bills and degradation of research atmosphere. It is proposed that honorarium be provided to researcher, as a parentage of the project fund. This percentage should be low for projects that have large expenses. On the other hand, this honorarium can be as higher for theoretical projects.

Patents

In research institutes of India, patents automatically belong to institutes (eg. IIT). Why should it be like this? The logic behind this is not clear. Despite the fact that the institutes claim that patents belong to the institute, the institute cannot file the patent without consent of the faculty inventor. One reason faculty meekly surrender this right is the high cost of filing the patent and maintaining it. Such patents rarely brings in income to the institute. Leaving aside exceptional cases, most of the patents are filed for prestige or promotion purpose. In fact, the institutes suffer huge financial burden to maintain these patents.

PARTICIPATION OF FACULTY IN ACTIVE POLITICS

Researchers, scholars and scientists usually have very fertile and creative brain. They have been advisor to the Kings and administrators all throughout the history. In many countries, such people are allowed to take active interest in politics, unlike India. Let us look at the following few cases:

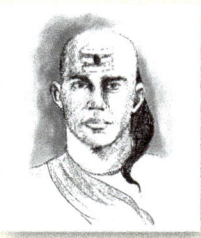

1. **Chanakya Kautilya:** He was originally a professor of economics and political science at the ancient university of Taxila. He has authored the book "Arthashastra" (Economics) and is considered as the pioneer of political science and classical economics. On the other hand, he assisted Mauryan Emperor Chandragupta to rise to power and later served as advisors to his successors Bindusara.

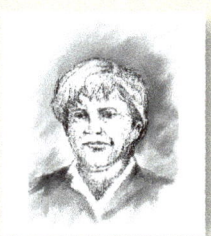

2. **Angela Dorothea Merkel,** is one of the most respected politician in Europe as the chancellor of Germany. She is considered as the voice of the European Union and is able to impact major decisions in the world today. But to start with, she studied physics at the University of Leipzig, earning a doctorate in 1978, and later worked as a chemist at the Central Institute for Physical Chemistry, Academy of Sciences .

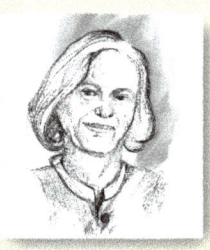

3. **Johanna Wanka** is the Federal Minister of Education an Secondary School in Grobtreben and the advanced school in Torgau before studying mathematics at Leipzig University in the GDR. She received her doctorate from Merseburg University of Applied Sciences and later became professor and Rector here.

The Madras High Court bench has held that government employees could be prohibited from being members of political parties and it would not amount to denying their fundamental rights. Dismissing a writ petition by an employee of Civil Supplies Department Justice S. Nagamuthu said "such prohibition will come under the purview of reasonable restrictions imposed on the fundamental rights." Though a person could not be denied entry into government service on the sole ground that he was involved in active politics, he could not be allowed to continue it after taking up government jobs.

This rule is usually extended to faculty in universities as they are Government Employee. But is this logic really Valid? Faculty should be allowed to participate in active politics under following conditions:
a. Public demonstration, disturbing the educational atmosphere should be discouraged.
b. Faculty should be allowed to interact with political parties and advice them, as long as their own professional activities are not affected.
c. Faculty should be allowed to take active participation in politics on deputation and rejoin institute within reasonable time frame.

RESEARCH PORTAL

The basic objective of this research portal is to promote and support transparency and public participation in research at national level, which is the need of present society. The present research culture needs drastic changes:

• Creation of a public demand driven portal, for researchers, public, institutes and private/public agencies and organizations.

• In order to participate in this portal, researcher must publish their output in video format visible through mobile and computer technology so that public can access, rate and provide financial support to the researcher. This support would include necessary expense for future research, institute component and honorarium. The researcher can also publish their future proposals and demonstrate their output in video format visible through mobile and computer technology. The publication will be peer reviewed.

• The general public and intellectuals would be able to select and float new topics on the portal, more relevant with their needs and requirement and which will be opened to voting, rating and sponsorship.

• A Rating system created for each proposed topics for research, will be based upon the number of votes and the monetary support pledged for the topics.

• Private company and government can use these indexes of ratings to provide financial support topic wise or to promising individual researchers.

• This will make researchers carry out research for the benefit of society as they are being monitored.

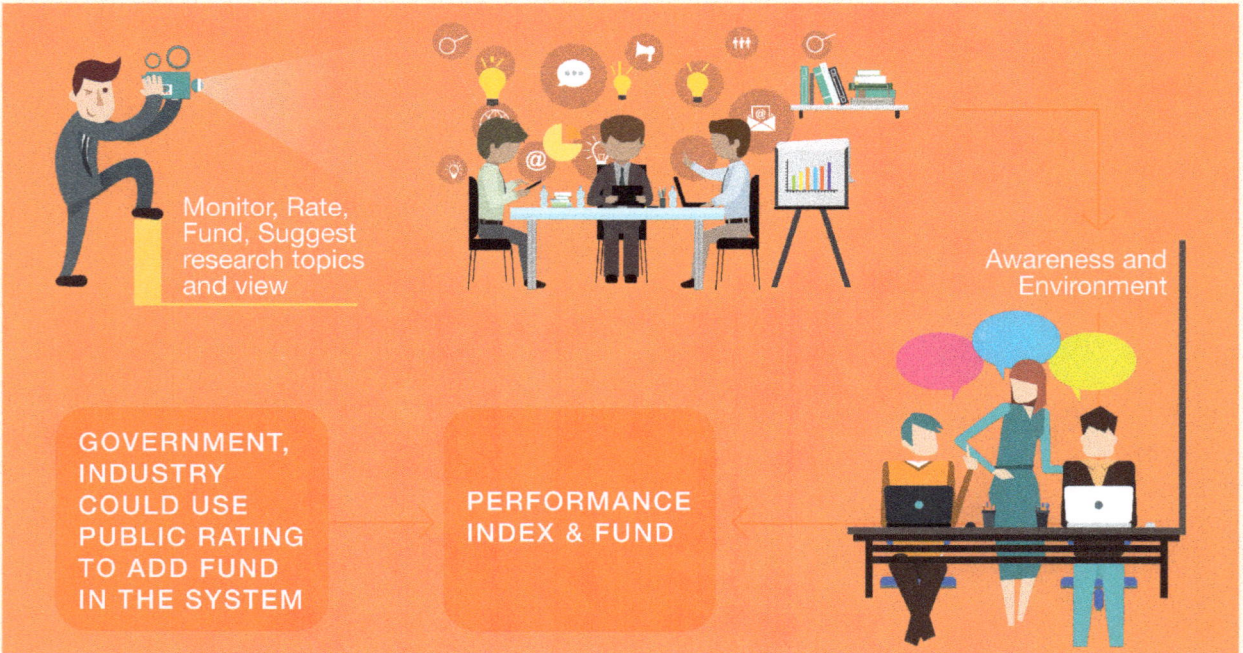

Monitor, Rate, Fund, Suggest research topics and view

Awareness and Environment

GOVERNMENT, INDUSTRY COULD USE PUBLIC RATING TO ADD FUND IN THE SYSTEM

PERFORMANCE INDEX & FUND

Print information available on the last page

To order additional copies of this book, contact
Partridge India
000 800 10062 62
www.partridgepublishing.com/india
orders.india@partridgepublishing.com

09/22/2016

PARTRIDGE